Herbal Remedies

A Guide to Herbal Remedies, Natural Remedies, Antivirals, Antibiotics and Alternative Medicine!

Table of Contents

Introduction 5

Chapter 1: Understanding Herbal Medicine 7

Chapter 2: The History of Herbal Medicine 11

Chapter 3: Creating Herbal Medicine 15

Chapter 4: Where to Find Herbal Medicine 18

Chapter 5: A List of Common Ailments and Their Treatments.. 22

Chapter 6: Commonly Used Healing Herbs 27

Chapter 7: Herbal Antibiotic Remedies 30

Chapter 8: Antiviral Herbal Remedies.................................. 33

Chapter 9: Herbal Remedies that Improve the Metabolism and Increase Energy.. 36

Chapter 10: Herbal Remedies to Combat Depression 38

Chapter 11: Using Herbal Supplements Safely 41

Conclusion 45

© Copyright 2016 - All rights reserved.

The follow eBook is reproduced below with the goal of providing information that is as accurate and reliable as possible. Regardless, purchasing this eBook can be seen as consent to the fact that both the publisher and the author of this book are in no way experts on the topics discussed within and that any recommendations or suggestions that are made herein are for entertainment purposes only. Professionals should be consulted as needed prior to undertaking any of the action endorsed herein.

This declaration is deemed fair and valid by both the American Bar Association and the Committee of Publishers Association and is legally binding throughout the United States.

Furthermore, the transmission, duplication or reproduction of any of the following work including specific information will be considered an illegal act irrespective of if it is done electronically or in print. This extends to creating a secondary or tertiary copy of the work or a recorded copy and is only allowed with express written consent from the Publisher. All additional right reserved.

The information in the following pages is broadly considered to be a truthful and accurate account of facts and as such any inattention, use or misuse of the information in question by the reader will render any resulting actions solely under their purview. There are no scenarios in which the publisher or the original author of this work can be in any fashion deemed liable for any hardship or damages that may befall them after undertaking information described herein.

Additionally, the information in the following pages is intended only for informational purposes and should thus be thought of as universal. As befitting its nature, it is presented without assurance regarding its prolonged validity or interim quality. Trademarks that are mentioned are done without written consent and can in no way be considered an endorsement from the trademark holder.

Introduction

Congratulations on picking up *Herbal Remedies: A Guide to Herbal Remedies, Natural Remedies, Antivirals, Antibiotics and Alternative Medicine!* and thank you for doing so. The fact of the matter is that pharmaceutical companies have long since passed the point where caring about patients is their number one priority. As lifesaving medicine grows ever higher in price, herbal remedies which have been around for generations once again are starting to seem like the best choice.

Despite its worldwide lineage stretching back beyond recorded history, herbal medicine has fallen by the wayside in many cultures in the past 200 years. To counteract that fact, the following chapters will explain everything you need to know in order to start getting the maximum benefits from any herbal remedies that you do choose to utilize. You will then find an abridged version of the history of herbal medicine, dating back to ancient China and ancient Egypt. From there you will learn about the various ways to create herbal medicine as well as where to find herbal alternatives near you.

You will then find chapters on numerous common ailments as well as herbs to treat them, the most commonly used healing herbs, herbs that are known to be high in antibiotics, herbs that are antiviral, herbal remedies for curing exhaustion and improving the metabolism, and herbal ways to deal with depression. Finally, you will learn the best ways to ensure, above all else, that you always use herbal supplements in a fashion that is as safe as possible.

There are plenty of books on this subject on the market, thanks again for choosing this one! Every effort was made to ensure it is full of as much useful information as possible, please enjoy!

Chapter 1:
Understanding Herbal Medicine

At its most basic, herbal medicine, also known as botanical medicine or herbalism, is the use of any plant, part of a plant, or herb, that is used expressly for its medicinal or therapeutic value, including treating current ailments or preventing new illnesses from developing. Despite the relatively recent popularity of Western medicine, herbal medicine is still the most commonly practiced type of medicine worldwide, just as it has been since time immemorial.

Currently, estimates put the use of herbal remedy products as a multi-billion dollar per year industry in the United States, with a majority of this coming from over the counter options to treat self-diagnosed problems. This is in line with modern herbalism which often slots specific types of herbal remedies into specific systems of the body.

Despite its ancient roots, modern science is often just catching up to what some cultures have never forgotten, that using a variety of herbs and spices is a healthy way to prevent disease in a wide variety of forms. While herbalists, those who deal in herbal remedies, are not licensed in the United States, there are numerous herbal remedies that are recommended on a regular basis in the form of tablets, capsules, tinctures and extracts for countless different medical conditions.

While the phrase 'herbal remedy' often conjures up visions of dietary supplements sold at most grocery stores, the truth of the matter is that a surprising number of common medicines are based on herbal standards. Not only does this mean that there are natural alternatives to numerous common medicines, often with fewer side effects, it also means that before you start taking anything discussed in the following pages you should take the time to determine if it is going to negatively interact with anything else you are currently taking.

Basic principles of herbal remedies

Goal of restoring balance to the body: Western medicine typically starts the diagnosis process by looking at individual symptoms and prescribing treatments that have worked for others in the past in combating the presumed disease. On the other hand, herbal medicine starts by looking at the person, not the symptoms, to determine lifestyle influences that can be adding undue physical stressors to the body, that are then actually the cause of the issue in question. This, in turn, allows an appropriate treatment to be prescribed that aims to get to the heart of the actual issue in question. Once the root of the problem has been determined, the right herbal treatment can then be recommended to help restore the balance to the body that has been lost.

Straight from the source: Many Western medicines, especially those that fall into the category of over the counter medicines, like to advertise that they are using natural ingredients in their products. The truth of the matter is they are often using what are known as active ingredients, or bits and pieces of the natural ingredient instead of the related plant as a whole, which can lead to side effects that are not present when the plant is consumed in full. A good example of this is salicylic acid, one of aspirin's active ingredients. If you have a sensitive stomach and take aspirin, then the salicylic acid is likely going to cause you some discomfort. However, if you take meadowsweet for the same issue, instead, then you won't have an issue as the mucilage and tannin that the meadowsweet contains neutralizes the negative affect the salicylic acid has on your stomach.

Secondary benefits: While various plants and herbs have different primary benefits, they all share a number of secondary benefits as well. First and foremost, they are easy to add into your daily dietary routine in numerous different ways, and can be grown at home making it extremely easy to get into the habit of improving your overall health. They are also applicable in a wide variety of situations, regardless if you are combating a chronic disease or some simple burns or scrapes. They are also useful when it comes to numerous different persistent illnesses including things like PMS, depression, arthritis, and migraines.

Herbal remedies compared to pharmaceuticals

Progression of treatment: Herbalists typically focus on treating the full person as it is believed that the illness that is currently presenting itself is only doing so because the body is currently out of alignment. This makes the goal of the herbalist to then restore balance and stimulate the body's natural ability to heal via positive changes to lifestyle and diet, and the addition of relevant herbal remedies. By contrast, Western medicine typically uses a more aggressive approach on the disease as presented, attacking it with the help of strong drugs and chemicals that can be worse on the body than the disease itself. If things don't improve, Western medicine often resorts to removing the infected area.

Makeup of the medicine: In the late 1980s, nearly 90 percent of all Western medicine drugs were still made from the active ingredients found in plants. Cut to 2016, and that number has fallen all the way to a mere 15 percent. These man-made elements are naturally more difficult for the body to metabolize, leading to an increase in side effects. On the other hand, herbal remedies are all natural, obviously, which typically makes them safer to use and easier for the body to handle, while at the same time leaving them less open to the chance that your body will not react as well regarding side effects. Essentially, certain remedies will work better for you than others while some will work worse.

Additionally, before you commit to a purely herbal remedy route, it is important to keep in mind that various factors, including things like the severity of the condition, the length of time that it has plagued you, and the method in which you choose to administer the treatment are all going to play a part in how long it might take for the issue to dissipate. This can be a short period of time, such as the minute or so it takes for herbal bitters to help with bloating or gas, a period of many months such as what is required to repair intense imbalances, or it could even take years for chronic or other serious conditions to reverse themselves.

Chapter 2:
The History of Herbal Medicine

While many people in the United States are just finding out about the wide variety of benefits that are possible with herbal remedies, the fact of the matter is that they have been a major part of the evolution of medicine dating back to the ancient Egyptians and beyond. In fact, scrolls dating back to 3,000 BC have been found in both China and Egypt describing plants as part of the healing process.

Ancient History: One of the oldest herbs in history is the popular ginkgo biloba. Fossil records show that Ginkgo has been on earth at least since the Paleozoic period. The first known recorded herbal study was written around 2,000 BC by the Chinese Emperor Shen Nong, called the *Shennong Bencaojing*. Nong is remembered for his dedication to seed preservation, dietary revolution and for the fact that he personally tasted over 300 herbs. The document that bears his name contains descriptions and information for more than 300 plants.

Some 500 years later, around 1500 BC, the Egyptians created one of the oldest surviving records of medical documents, called papyrus ebers. This long scroll documents 700 plant-based remedies. During the middle ages, monks also grew medicinal herbs. The liquor Bénédictine was made at the Benedictine Abbey of Fecamp in Normandy with 27 different plants and spices and its restorative properties were often attributed to a higher power.

Native Americans introduced the colonists to plants and herbs such as black cohosh, which is still used today for relieving menstrual cramps and menopause symptoms. In fact, the

American College of Obstetricians and Gynecologists officially recognizes the value of black cohosh.

Modern day: The modern era began in the 1800s when scientists first gained access to the field of chemical analysis. This practice allowed them to begin extracting, and eventually modifying, the active ingredients they discovered in their traditional herbal remedies. Starting in the 1900s, innovations in chemical analysis allowed scientists to extract and modify active ingredients from plants. Some of the most effective medicines of the time include aspirin (made using willow bark), morphine (made from certain types of poppies), quinine (made from cinchona bark) and digoxin (made from foxglove).

In America, clashes within the medical community and a growing infatuation with isolated chemicals led to the decline of herbal remedies over the years. However, even today new pharmaceutical drugs are based on botanicals and the twenty-first century has seen a resurgence of interest in herbal alternatives to caustic manmade medicines.

Despite the overall decline of plant matter in Western medicine, the World Health Organization stipulates that more than 80 percent of the population of the world still uses herbal medicines as part of their main health care habits. Of particular note in this instance, is Germany, where more than 600 different types of herbal remedies are currently prescribed by more than 70 percent of the country's physicians.

East versus West

One interesting fact about herbal remedies is the fact that they are often considered so universal. In fact, regardless of where you go in the world you are likely to find locals using variations of the same plants and herbs to treat the same illnesses. Nevertheless, two different philosophies have developed over time, Eastern herbalism and Western herbalism.

Western herbalism: Western herbalism can trace its roots all the way back to ancient Egypt when juniper as well as garlic were used to treat various ailments. These early concepts were codified over time until the ancient Greeks were able to use them to develop a philosophy regarding herbal medicine that is still considered fairly comprehensive. It includes delineations related to seasons and temperaments; as well as the elements water, fire, air and earth, each of which was considered a classification of various types of ailments. This philosophy was further expanded upon by the Romans, creating the basis of the modern medical philosophy that is still in use today.

Eastern herbalism: On the other hand, herbalism in the Eastern tradition is believed to come from a mix of Ayurveda teachings as well as those that are considered Chinese medicine in the more traditional sense. The combination of these two is used to allow the body to restore balance to itself naturally. In Chinese herbalism, the Qi (energy) and the dual concepts of yin and yang all play a part. In this practice, each type of herb is noted to be in possession of certain qualities. Those that are said to have cooling qualities are associated with yin and those that ae said to have stimulating qualities are associated with yang. They are then used in various different combinations as needed to restore the user's Qi to its desired levels.

Chapter 3:
Creating Herbal Medicine

Before you go ahead and start self-diagnosing all of your problems based on the herbal remedies you have access to, it is important to remember that just because the effects from natural versions of common medicines are going to be milder than the chemical versions, doesn't mean that they should be used over-enthusiastically as they can still have negative results if treated recklessly. This means you are going to want to consult a medical text or a professional on the matter before you dive into it in full force.

It is important to keep in mind that herbal supplements can be consumed as a liquid, capsule, or powder, and in their natural state either chopped, dried, or even raw. This variety of states is akin to the variety of different ways they can affect individuals which means when you are first getting started it is important to take things slowly until you know how your body is going to react to the things you are putting in it.

What's more, if you seek out a place to buy herbal remedies without doing your homework, you often won't be able to rely on labels to help you as many types of remedies are not allowed to advertise what they treat specifically. As an example, St. John's wort is often cited as a viable way to naturally treat ongoing feelings of depression. While this has been known to be the case for hundreds of years, modern labels on bottle of St. John's wort can only legally say it enhances mood. Do yourself a favor, know what it is you are looking for before you start looking in order to ensure you get the best results from your search.

While many studies show that various herbal remedies are effective at treating the ailments they are attributed with aiding, the exact reason as to why they do so is typically still a mystery. This is because it is difficult for scientists to determine when certain active ingredients are working alone and when they are reacting to various other elements in the herb in question. Furthermore, certain herbs are known to be more or less effective based on the location they were grown in, as well as how they were processed or harvested, making nailing down specifics extra tricky.

Creating herbal remedies

Tincture: Tinctures are created by placing herbs in a mixture of alcohol and water with the ultimate goal being to preserve as well as extract any active ingredients the herbs might possess. This liquid is then cured for a prolonged period of time and then taken at regular intervals by placing drops of it on the tongue.

Creams: Creams are typically made from a mixture that is comprised of fat or oils, as well as herbs. The combination is them simmered for at least three hours before being strained and bottled.

Ointment: Ointments are typically made from a mixture that is comprised of fat or oils, as well as herbs. Unlike creams which are simmered, the ingredients for ointments are heated with a quickness using boiling water, before being strained and then set immediately.

Decoction: A decoction is made in the same manner as an ointment, by extracting essential ingredients via boiling, except that instead of herbs it uses a mixture of berries, roots and barks. The results are then strained and consumed either hot or cold, depending on the particulars.

Infusion: An infusion is made in much the same way that tea is made. Specifically, the herb is placed in a container before being submerged in steaming liquid and allowed to steep anywhere from 15 minutes to several hours. Infusions are best consumed hot in small doses. An infusion can either be made with water or with oil. To make your own infusion you are going to want to place the herbs of your choice into a canning jar, before then filling the jar with either oil or water. Steep as desired before straining out the herbs after the liquid has cooled. In a 16-ounce jar, three handfuls of herbs should suffice for an average potency.

Chapter 4:
Where to Find Herbal Medicine

While you can easily find a wide variety of herbal remedies of all sorts everywhere from online to your local gas station, the fact of the matter is that it is still best to talk to a professional before you start putting anything into your body on the regular. An herbalist, or at least a person who works at an herbal supplement or remedy store should at least be able to point you in the right direction, and maybe even help treat the issue behind what is causing the symptoms in the first place.

Herbal remedy stores

When you visit a modern herbal supplement or remedy store you are likely going to have access to a wide variety of processed or partially processed herbs, typically in either the form of already made tinctures, extracts, oils, syrups, teas, capsules, and pills. Teas can be made from either powders or dried herbs, while syrups can also be added to cold or hot water to form an on the go infusion. Oils can be useful either as part of a food, your own cream or ointment, or even as the base for an exceptionally rejuvenating massage.

The tinctures that you find in stores are generally going to be a single part herb, and anywhere from 10 parts to 5 parts liquid, with the smaller amount of liquid directly equating to a more potent tincture. If you come across what is known as a liquid extract, be aware that is not the same, and is in fact much more potent than a standard tincture. Specifically, liquid extracts contain a single part of the herbal remedy in question and also a single part liquid making them anywhere from 5 to ten 10 as strong as a traditional tincture. Finally, you may come across dry extracts which come in capsule, tablet or lozenge form and are even more potent than the liquid extracts, containing anywhere from 2 to 8 parts herbal remedy to a single part liquid.

Don't forget, the products that these stores sell are in no way regulated which means that when it comes to looking for a store to frequent on the regular, what you are going to want to do is to choose one which offers a guarantee on its products irrespective of where they come from. Additionally, you will want to ensure that the staff of the store that you choose are knowledgeable of the products that they sell, and can help you with dosing specifications when you decide to try something new. Above all, you are going to want to ensure that the store you visit puts off a professional, low pressure vibe, as for every herbal remedy that actually works there are 4 on the market that are essentially snake oil and you want to trust that what you are buying will actually help with its intended purpose.

Find an herbalist

While seeking out a local herbal remedy store is a great choice to help you decide if treating ailments with herbal solutions is right for you, if you do find that you want to explore the herbal possibilities more completely, you are going to want to seek out your own person herbalist instead. An herbalist is someone who has spent years, if not decades, studying the types of plants that you are gaining an interest in and can include anyone from herb farmers, wild crafters, medicine makers, pharmacists, researcher, naturopaths, native healers, and holistic doctors, just to name but a few. These individuals can then either practice their trade as consultants or as full on primary healthcare providers.

The first consultation: When it comes to choosing an herbalist that is right for you, the first step is to do some research and find a few options that appeal to you in your local area. It is important to keep positive and negative reviews in mind and look for the truth that is at the heart of any review bias.

Once you know where you want to start, the next thing you are going to want to do is to schedule a consultation to allow you and the herbalist you fancy to meet one another, and to allow the herbalist to get a feel for your history as well as your lifestyle, dietary choices, and anything else that might be negatively affecting your overall health. The consultation will typically end with the herbalist coming up with a rough outline of a personalized health program that would be implemented if you choose to move forward. The goal here is to treat the entire individual, not just one disease which is just a symptom of a larger issue.

Types of herbalists to consider: Various herbalists are going to follow different variations of the same practices, depending on what type of tradition that they adhere to. There are numerous different types of herbalist practices including Native American herbal traditions, Chinese medicine, Ayurveda, naturopathic medicine, and Western herbal medicine to name a few. Different types of herbalists are all going to recommend different variations of treatment which means that you are going to want to do more than read reviews, you are going to want to read up on the various types of herbalists as well.

Western herbalists are known to base their treatments on the historical and traditional treatments that have been passed down since the days of the ancient Greeks. These days they are often trained at traditional schools and universities and many spend almost as long in training as a more traditional doctor.

This training includes a detailed study of anatomy, nutrition, biochemistry, medical science, and more.

Naturopathic herbalists are known to integrate a mix of western medical standards, up to date medical diagnoses, and natural therapeutic solutions into their work. If you visit a licensed naturopathic doctor, then you know that they have received medical training at an accredited university akin to any more traditional doctor. Only 13 states currently allow licensed individuals to practice naturopathy.

Ayurvedic medicine is a practice that comes from the area surrounding Nepal and India, and is one of the most popular types of herbal medicine on the planet today, with more than 80 percent of Indians regularly seeing a Ayurvedic doctor. These individuals attend school for 12 years to practice their skills. In the United States, you are going to want to look for an Ayurvedic doctor that has the title M.D. Ayur, and also has an accreditation from the American Ayurvedic Association.

Outside of Western medicine, traditional Chinese medicine is the most frequently cited medical system in the world. Doctors who practice this type of herbalism study extensively to learn acupuncture, herbal therapy and the practice and theory of herbalism in all its forms. Many states officially license acupuncturists and many types of insurance allow for visits to this type of herbalist as well.

Chapter 5:
A List of Common Ailments and Their Treatments

Acne: Common herbal remedy treatments are known to include - Tea tree, aloe vera and calendula

Alcoholism: Common herbal remedy treatments are known to include - Kudzu and evening primrose

Allergies: Common herbal remedy treatments are known to include - Chamomile

Angina: Common herbal remedy treatments are known to include - Willow, garlic and green tea

Anxiety: Common herbal remedy treatments are known to include - Chamomile, passionflower, kava and lavender

Arthritis: Common herbal remedy treatments are known to include - Cat's claw, devil's claw, turmeric and ginger

Asthma: Common herbal remedy treatments are known to include - Tea, ephedra and coffee

Athletes foot: Common herbal remedy treatments are known to include - Tea tree oil

Bad breath: Common herbal remedy treatments are known to include - Parsley

Boils: Common herbal remedy treatments are known to include - Ginseng, Echinacea, topical garlic, tea tree oil

Bronchitis: Common herbal remedy treatments are known to include - Pelargonium, Echinacea

Burns: Common herbal remedy treatments are known to include - Aloe

Canker Sores: Common herbal remedy treatments are known to include - Goldenseal

Colds: Common herbal remedy treatments are known to include - Coffee, licorice root, ginseng, Echinacea

Constipation: Common herbal remedy treatments are known to include - Senna, psyllium seed, apple

Cough: Common herbal remedy treatments are known to include - Eucalyptus

Depression: Common herbal remedy treatments are known to include - St. John's wort

Diarrhea: Common herbal remedy treatments are known to include – Raspberry and bilberry

Dizziness: Common herbal remedy treatments are known to include – Ginkgo balboa and ginger

Earache: Common herbal remedy treatments are known to include – Echinacea

Fatigue: Common herbal remedy treatments are known to include – Rhodiola, ginseng, coffee, cocoa

Flu: Common herbal remedy treatments are known to include – Elderberry, Echinacea

Gas: Common herbal remedy treatments are known to include – Dill and fennel

Gingivitis: Common herbal remedy treatments are known to include – Green Tea and goldenseal

Hay fever: Common herbal remedy treatments are known to include – Butterbur and stinging nettle

Herpes: Common herbal remedy treatments are known to include – Garlic, ginger, topical comfrey, topical lemon balm

High blood pressure: Common herbal remedy treatments are known to include – Hawthorn, garlic

High blood sugar: Common herbal remedy treatments are known to include – fenugreek

High cholesterol: Common herbal remedy treatments are known to include – Primrose oil, flax seed, cinnamon and apple

Hot flashes: Common herbal remedy treatments are known to include – black cohosh, soy, and red clover

Impotence: Common herbal remedy treatments are known to include – Yohimbe

Indigestion: Common herbal remedy treatments are known to include – Peppermint, ginger, and chamomile

Infection: Common herbal remedy treatments are known to include – Garlic, Echinacea, astragals, tea tree oil

Insomnia: Common herbal remedy treatments are known to include – Valerian, lemon balm, evening primrose, kava

Lower back pain: Common herbal remedy treatments are known to include – While willow bark, carvacrol and thymol

Menstrual cramps: Common herbal remedy treatments are known to include – Chasteberry, Raspberry and kava

Migraine: Common herbal remedy treatments are known to include – Butterbur and feverfew

Morning sickness: Common herbal remedy treatments are known to include – Ginger

Muscle pain: Common herbal remedy treatments are known to include – Wintergreen and capsicum

Seasonal affective disorder: Common herbal remedy treatments are known to include – St. John's Wort

Shingles: Common herbal remedy treatments are known to include – Capsicum

Sore throat: Common herbal remedy treatments are known to include – Mullein, marshmallow and licorice

Stuffy nose: Common herbal remedy treatments are known to include – Echinacea

Tonsillitis: Common herbal remedy treatments are known to include – Astragals, Echinacea and goldenseal

Toothache: Common herbal remedy treatments are known to include – Clove oil and willow

Ulcers: Common herbal remedy treatments are known to include – Licorice and aloe

Varicosities: Common herbal remedy treatments are known to include – Horse chestnut and bilberry

Yeast infection: Common herbal remedy treatments are known to include – goldenseal and garlic

Chapter 6:
Commonly Used Healing Herbs

The healing herbs that are outlined below have been used to treat every malady under the sun for millennia. If you have a minor illness, ache or pain, the following herbs are all a good place to start.

Aloe: This herb is commonly used topically to treat skin inflammation, irritation, sunburn, and other mild burns

Arnica: This herb is commonly used topically to treat sore joints, sore muscles, minor sprains, and serious bruising

Chamomile: This herb is commonly used in tea as a way of treating colic, indigestion, heartburn, and upset stomach

Comfrey: This herb is commonly used in a poultice to treat spider bites, ulcers that are caused by diabetes, staph infections, and bedsores

Dongquai: This herb is commonly used in tonics as a means for women to improve their overall stamina and general health

Echinacea: This herb is commonly used to treat the symptoms of a sore throat, the flu, and even the common cold

Evening primrose oil: This herb is commonly used to treat endometriosis, breast pain, menopause symptoms, premenstrual syndrome, acne, eczema, and other skin disorders

Feverfew: This herb is commonly used to treat migraine headaches

Garlic: This herb is commonly used to treat the common cold, fungal infections, high blood pressure, and reduce cholesterol

Ginger: This herb is commonly used to treat motion sickness, nausea, and is generally prized for its anti-inflammatory properties

Ginkgo biloba: This herb is commonly used to as a way to promote antioxidants in the blood stream, as well as an overall healthy brain

Ginseng: This herb is commonly used to treat sexual dysfunction issues and diabetes, while also providing excess energy, reduced blood sugar, and lowered stress levels.

Goldenseal: This herb is commonly used to treat vaginitis, digestive issues, eye infections, allegories, respiratory infections, as well as to help promote healthy skin, and reduce the risk of cancer

Milk thistle: This herb is commonly used to treat various issues associated with the liver, typically found in alcoholics and those with AIDS

Mullein: This herb is commonly used to treat coughing related to bronchitis, as well as general chest congestion

Passionflower: This herb is commonly used as a way to provide a relaxed state that is not based on a sedative

Peppermint oil: When ingested in capsules, this herb is commonly used to treat digestive problems, nausea, indigestion, irritable bowel syndrome, and other similar ailments

Saw palmetto: This herb is commonly used to treat hair loss, and is also known to benefit the prostate

Tea tree oil: This herb is commonly used to treat fungal infections that start underneath the fingernails and toenails, as well as the fungal infection that causes athlete's foot

Turmeric: This herb is commonly used to ward off inflammation, and is also believed to ward off Alzheimer's disease and cancer

Valerian: This herb is commonly used to treat sleep related issues

Chapter 7:
Herbal Antibiotic Remedies

Many different herbs are prized for their ability to provide antibiotic protection against a host of ailments. The list is outlined in detail below.

Butterbur: Very popular in Europe, this herb, which has recently entered the American market, contains petasines, an herbal mixture which quells inflammation and allergic response, just as effectively as Allegra and Zyrtec, according to recent studies.

Calendula: This herb is commonly used to treat pink eye; it is also known to help to prevent overall infection and to help wounds heal more quickly. Calendula has no known required precautions and can easily be added to ointments, lotions, tinctures, and infusions.

Cinnamon sticks: This spice is commonly used to help the digestive process and is also known to have numerous antibacterial properties. It can be ingested as a supplement, taken with food, or brewed in a tea. All methods are equally effective.

Clove: In its base form, clove is known to be a useful analgesic because it naturally numbs affected areas, and when dried it is also useful when it comes to preventing harmful intestinal bacteria from multiplying. Adding dried clove to tea tends to offer the best antibacterial results.

Garlic: This potent herb is known to treat a variety of different bacterial strains more effectively than penicillin does. What's more, it is also much less caustic to the system because it attacks the bacteria in question, while leaving beneficial intestinal flora unharmed, something that can't be said of penicillin. Garlic is believed to be most beneficial when consumed in a concentrated capsule or tincture, though it will still benefit you if you add more of it to your diet as long as you don't heat it past 125 degrees to avoid decreasing its potency.

Goldenseal: This herb is known to promote healthy skin, prevent colds, reduce the risk of respiratory infections, improve allergy symptoms, reduce eye infections, improve digestive issues, mitigate vaginitis, and help reduce the risk of cancer.

Echinacea: While it can be harmful to those with autoimmune diseases, it is known to noticeably increase healing time when taken regularly via tincture.

Oregon grape root: This antibacterial herb is known to be especially effective when taken in conjunction with Echinacea. It is best taken via tincture though not for a prolonged period of time as then it is known to reduce the rate at which the body can absorb Vitamin B. Oregon grape root should not be taken by those who have glaucoma, hypertension, or a history or increased risk of stroke or diabetes. It should also not be taken by women who are pregnant or currently breastfeeding.

Marshmallow root: This herb is known for its pain reducing qualities as well as for the fact that it can minimize scarring and improve healing time. It is also known to contain tannins which are especially effective when it comes to fighting bacteria that attack the urinary tract. Marshmallow root is believed to be most effective when brewed into a tea.

Stinging Nettle: While it may seem counterintuitive, the leaves of the stinging nettle plant are known to be extremely effective when it comes to combating allergy symptoms of all sorts.

Usnea: No so much an herb as it is a lichen, usnea is known to be both antifungal and antibacterial, in addition to being a powerful antibiotic in its own right. It is often used to help treat and prevent vaginosis, yeast infections, fungal infections, sinus infections, respiratory infections, staph infections, and strep infections, primarily in a tincture form. Women who are pregnant are recommended to consult an herbalist prior to use.

Uva Ursi: This herb is frequently used for treating severe urinary tract infections and is known to target pathogens that target the urinary tract. It is primarily taken as a capsule or a tincture, and because of this high concentration should only be used in 2 week stretches. Those who are suffering from kidney disease, children, and women who are pregnant or nursing should not take uva ursi.

Yarrow: This tiny flower is useful when powdered as it can help cuts close more quickly. When it is properly infused in water it is also know to improve the rate at which canker sores heal, and if it is brewed into a tea it strengthens the urinary tract and prevents against infection. Women who are pregnant should avoid yarrow as it is known to cause contractions.

Chapter 8:
Antiviral Herbal Remedies

Many different herbs are prized for their ability to provide antiviral protection against a host of ailments. The list is outlined in detail below.

Astragalus root: This root is known to help prevent viral infections regardless if it is consumed via tincture, capsule, or even as part of a soup or stew. It not only helps you overall, it immensely boosts your immune system for a few hours after consumption, so it is a great choice before dealing with crowds during periods of increased illness. However, it can exacerbate a fever if you already have it before taking the astragalus root, so it is best to lay off if you are already ill.

Cat's Claw: Cat's claw is an herb that is a triple threat, it is antiviral, antifungal, and antibacterial as well. It is also known to increase the body's natural resistance to all sort of illnesses regardless if it consumed via capsule, tincture, or tea. It should be avoided by women who are currently pregnant.

Cranberry: When concentrated, the simple cranberry becomes more than a delicious Thanksgiving treat. It provides a powerful defense against urinary tract infections. It works by making the bladder too slippery for invading viruses to latch on to. Cranberries are also high in antioxidants, and are even known to help prevent plaque from building up on teeth when consumed in their unsweetened berry form. Otherwise, a concentrated capsule is likely going to be your best bet.

Elderberry: The elderberry is commonly used to bolster the immune system in the midst of either cold or flu symptoms. They are also known to help cleanse the body of negative toxins, and also cause sweating whilst improving circulation. Syrup is the most common elderberry delivery method, and during periods of infection everyone is encouraged to consume up to 3 tablespoons each day. It is important to only ingest the syrup, as the berries, seeds, roots, and leaves are all known to be poisonous and even contain cyanide.

Ginger root: When dried, ginger root is known to have strong antibacterial as well as antiviral properties, which means it is ideal when it comes to fighting off the common cold more quickly than otherwise might be possible. It is equally potent regardless if it is consumed in a capsule, via tea, or as an ingredient in any meal.

Lemon leaf balm: This balm is known to contain antiviral properties and specifically aids the digestive system and soothes an upset stomach, while at the same time instilling a feeling of calm. It is best consumed powdered and brewed into a tea. Women who are pregnant should consult an herbalist prior to use.

Licorice root: While it might flavor a classic type of candy, licorice root is also known to be both antibacterial and antiviral, and is often called into play as a way to repair gastric ulcers by attacking the virus that causes them, without upsetting the damaged stomach lining any more than it has already been damaged. For best results you are going to want to steep the root into a tea, though it should be avoided by women who are currently pregnant.

Mullein: When it is infused into an oil, mullein is a great way to clear up a variety of ear problems, including chronic ear infections. It is especially potent when it is combined with garlic and they are both infused into an oil together.

Olive leaf: The olive leaf has antiviral properties that run the gamut when it comes to common treatments as it is used for everything from the common cold, to the flu, to even herpes. It is effective as a tea, capsule, or tincture, and is especially effective when combined with mint. Women who are pregnant should avoid olive leaf in all its forms.

Oregano leaf: Not just a cooking herb, oregano is actually known to protect against bacteria and viruses, and is one of the most potent antiviral herbs you can find! Its capsule form is typically the most potent because cooking often saps it of its nutritional value.

Chapter 9:
Herbal Remedies that Improve the Metabolism and Increase Energy

Many different herbs are prized for their ability to provide a boost to the metabolism, or other types of feelings of increased energy. The list is outlined in detail below.

Alpha lipoic acid (ALA): This is an antioxidant supplement that is a great way to speed up metabolic reactions in the body, increasing energy production in the process. It does this by acting as an enzyme which reacts to the B-vitamins that are already in your system, supercharging them.

Co-enzyme (Q10): This enzyme also improves the production rate of energy that cells output. Studies show that this supplement generally increases overall vigor, and tolerance for physical strain as well.

Evening primrose oil: Studies show that taking anywhere between 500 mg and 1,000 mg of evening primrose oil each day will add crucial fatty acids missing from many diets into your system. This, in turn, is known to do wonders in a majority of individuals who are suffering from prolonged feelings of fatigue.

Guarana: The supplement known as guarana is actually a combination of several different types of natural stimulants which include guaranine, which is similar in effect to caffeine though it is released slowly into the body throughout the day. As a whole, guarana is known to reduce feelings of fatigue, increase energy levels, and temporarily improve alertness.

Kelp: More than just a type of seaweed, kelp is an extremely nutritious plant that contains numerous vital amino acids, as well as minerals and vitamins. Powdered kelp is typically consumed as an iodine supplement and by those looking to maintain a steadier overall level of energy throughout the day. Kelp should only be taken under the recommendation or supervision of an herbalist.

Magnesium: As many as 1 in 10 Americans is estimated to have a magnesium deficiency right now. This is a much more serious issue than it may appear, however, as magnesium is directly responsible for ensuring that more than 300 enzymes throughout the body continue to work at maximum efficiency. This includes key metabolic reactions such as keeping your metabolism running effectively, and generating energy from stored glucose. Those who have a magnesium deficiency may find themselves suffering from cramps, muscle spasms, weakness, fatigue, nausea, and a lack of appetite.

Siberian ginseng: Unlike its more common cousin, Siberian ginseng is what is known as an adaptogen, which means that is an ideal supplement during times of extreme stress or hardship as it improves both strength and stamina. It is also known to fight prolonged feelings of fatigue and aid in recovery.

Korean ginseng: This is one of the oldest known stimulant herbs in the world, it is also one of the oldest known sedatives - it all depends on what part of the plant is utilized in a tonic. If the smaller roots are used then they will create a tonic that is a sedative, if the central tap root is used instead, then it becomes a stimulant.

Chapter 10:
Herbal Remedies to Combat Depression

Depression comes in many different sizes and affects every individual in unique ways. While some types of depression will always be better off being treated with medication, there are others that respond positively to a whole host of herbal remedies which are outlined below.

Omega 3 fatty acids: Omega 3 fatty acids are a crucial component of continued healthy brain function. Omega 3 fatty acids are found in high amounts in fish, though capsules can also be purchased if you are afraid of consuming too much mercury. Among other things, omega 3s are known to be effective in helping those who are dealing with depression, and also in promoting weight loss. Omega 3 supplements are known to have interactions with several types of blood thinning drugs, including aspirin. Additionally, it should not be taken after surgery as it has been known to cause bleeding.

Sam-e: Short for, S-adenosyl-L-methionine, it is a chemical that should be naturally produced in the body, though some people's bodies don't naturally produce it in the amounts that are required. When it exists in appropriate amounts it improves the efficacy of the dopamine and serotonin that your body creates. It can be found in capsules at many health food stores, and is known to help fight osteoarthritis as well. It is, however, known to cause constipation and nausea in some cases.

Folic acid: Also known as folate, folic acid is a vitamin in the B vitamin family, and those who don't eat enough green vegetables are often going to be deficient in it. There are also several chronic conditions and medications, including birth control pills, that also lead to this deficiency.

5 HTTP: Also known as 5-hydroxytryptophan, this chemical is naturally produced by the body and is directly responsible for the creation of serotonin. 5 HTTP can boost the body's natural production of serotonin in some individuals. It should only be taken under doctor supervision and should not be mixed with most traditional antidepressants.

Vitamin B6: B6 is an important vitamin when it comes to the production of both dopamine and serotonin. While B6 is naturally produced inside the body, there are numerous oral contraceptives, drugs, and hormone replacement therapies that can cause an imbalance to occur.

Ginkgo biloba: In addition to benefitting the memory, ginkgo biloba is known to help treat or prevent specific circulatory disorders. It is also known to combat some types of depression, specifically among older individuals. As it is a blood thinner, those who are already taking blood thinners, those who have been known to have seizures, and those dealing with issues relating to fertility should discuss their plans with a doctor prior to use.

Kava kava: This herb is known to enhance feelings of relaxation, contentment, and wellbeing, while also elevating overall mood. It is also known to help treat numerous nervousness and anxiety disorders, though overuse can cause liver damage. While the specifics of the liver issues are not well-known, the product is still on the market in the United States, though it should only be taken under the supervision of a trained herbalist.

St. John's wort: This herb is commonly called upon for its anti-inflammatory and antidepressant properties. Numerous studies indicate that it is actually more effective than a placebo when it comes to treating anything up to and including moderate depression, with far fewer side effects than the drugs which behave in the same manner. It can take up to 6 weeks to infuse your system fully to the point where you notice a difference. Common side effects include fatigue, indigestion, dry mouth, and dizziness. It is also known to cause an increased sensitivity to sunlight in some people. Those who are already taking antidepressants should not start taking St. John's wort without consulting their prescribing physician.

Chapter 11:
Using Herbal Supplements Safely

When they are used properly, many herbal remedies can successfully treat a wide variety of issues, oftentimes better than more commonly used medications and almost always with fewer side effects. This does not mean that herbal remedies should be taken with disregard to personal safety as there are numerous scenarios where they could react negatively to existing medications or medical conditions.

Additionally, it is important to keep in mind that the herbal remedy market is largely unregulated, which means that when you first get ready to try a new brand or product, you are always going to want to do so with caution. This means that you are always going to want to follow dosage instructions to the letter, or even err on the side of caution to a small degree. Additionally, you are going to want to keep a close eye on exactly what you took, as well as the time you consumed it. This will not only allow you to tell if it has been effective, it will help you to give the details to a professional if you have a negative reaction.

FDA guidelines: Additionally, you will want to be aware that in the United States, the Federal Drug Administration classifies herbal remedies as either food or supplements, depending on the specifics of the remedy in question. This means that they are not regulated in the way that manmade drugs are, which means there is no standardization process when it comes to labeling, manufacturing, or even testing. Furthermore, they are not even required to guarantee a level of batch consistency, which means that certain pills can be more or less potent than the average. What all of this means is that you are going to need to do your homework on the various types of herbal remedies that interest you the most, and determine the most reliable version of each, as you never know what you are going to get if you grab a random brand off of the shelf.

However, this doesn't mean that manufactures can simply do anything they want - they will still have to ensure that their supplement regularly meets general quality standards. This means that products that you find on the shelf in larger stores should be as free of lead, pesticides, contaminants, and inaccurate ingredients as any other consumer product. Furthermore, after a supplement has been placed on the market, the FDA is then required to monitor it in a passive way. As such, if somewhere down the line the product is reported as being unsafe, then it is the FDA's job to go after the maker of the product and ensure that changes are made one way or another.

As such, these rules assure that products that are on shelves are going to be relatively safe to use in general, however it makes no claims as to the safety of any of the products in question in particular. Furthermore, this in no way applies to products that are purchased online, or products that herbal remedy stores have purchased via the same process. If you buy herbal remedy products online, ensure that you do plenty of research beforehand to ensure you are purchasing them through someone reputable.

Looking into specific herbal supplements: When it comes to determine what a specific herbal remedy is actually comprised of and whether or not it will really be good for you, the first thing that you are going to want to do is to look into the manufacturer as well as the distributor if possible. You will want to avoid the company website, and instead look for third party customer reviews or any news stories related to them. You will then want to check the name of the product in question, though this is subject to change, so assuming you find nothing of interest, or nothing at all, you will want to look into each of the ingredients. Assuming the ingredient list presents no red flags, you will want to ensure that the amount of each ingredient is acceptable. Assuming everything checks out, you can then take a recommended dose with confidence.

If you are having a hard time finding details on a specific ingredient, an herbalist is always going to be your best choice. Avoid seeking help at a local herbal supplement store as you will have no way of knowing if the employee was trying to make a sale or to actually tell you something useful. When it comes to comparing the labels of different herbal remedies, the easiest way to do so is by utilizing the Dietary Supplement Label Database, which can be found at the website for the National Institute of Health. This database can provide you with details on what's in all of the supplements currently on the market in the United States. Products can be searched for based on manufacturer, ingredient, brand, or even usage.

You are also going to want to be sure to regularly check the websites for both the NCCAM and the FDA to ensure that the supplements that you take on the regular haven't been added to the list that are currently under review. You will also want to keep an eye on the current list of supplements that are known to have adverse effects on those who take them in case any new issues have been recently found. While all of this might seem a tad excessive, it is better to do a little bit of homework than to risk accidentally doing more harm to yourself than good. Remember the old adage, an ounce of prevention is always going to be worth more than a pound of cure.

Verifying claims: Once you have a clear idea of what the various ingredients in the herbal supplement that you are considering actually do, you will already be well on your way to verifying any claims that the company who sells the product makes about what their product actually does. While these companies can't come right out and lie regarding their claims, it can be possible that their research was done in a way that would present results in their favor.

If your research hasn't provided you with a clear indication one way or another, the first thing you'll want to do is speak with a professional and have them weigh in on the topic. If that proves less than enlightening, the next place you will want to consider is the National Center for Complementary and Alternative Medicine (NCCAM), as well as the Office of Dietary Supplements. NCCAM provides a collection of studies that have been done by various supplement manufacturers, that allow you to see for yourself if the tests that were done were scientifically valid. The Office of Dietary Supplements also contains plenty of information compiled expressly to make it easier for consumers to make informed herbal choices.

Finally, if you remain unsatisfied, there is no reason that you shouldn't go ahead and give the manufacturer a call directly and see what type of information that they can provide you with. While the first person you speak with may not be able to answer all of your questions, if you can't eventually be connected with someone who can explain why the label makes the claims it does, then you should most likely find another supplement.

Conclusion

Thank for making it through to the end of *'Herbal Remedies: A Guide to Herbal Remedies, Natural Remedies, Antivirals, Antibiotics and Alternative Medicine!'*. I hope it was informative and able to provide you with all of the tools you need to achieve your goals, whatever it is that they may be. Just because you've finished this book doesn't mean there is nothing left to learn on the topic - expanding your horizons is the only way to find the mastery you seek.

Regardless of what personal issues you are currently dealing with, the fact of the matter is that there are currently several herbal remedies out there that can improve your overall quality of life. All that you need to do now is find them and find a brand that you can trust in order to provide you with a relatively reliable source of the herbal remedies that you have decided are right for you. When it comes to ensuring you get the most out of any herbal remedies you do choose to implement, it is important to first and foremost, not expect results overnight.

While certain products can offer results for specific issues in a short period of time, the truth of the matter is that many issues, especially those that fall on the more serious side of things, can take many weeks before you start to see results. In the interim, it is important that you keep the faith and keep up your herbal remedy treatments. Additionally, it has been said at several points in the preceding pages, but herbal remedies can often be quite potent which means that you are going to need to treat them with respect if you hope to get optimal results. Stick with the suggested dose, and don't underestimate what you are getting yourself into.

Finally, if you found this book useful in anyway, a review on Amazon is always appreciated!

CANCELLED

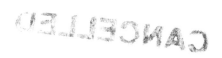

 CPSIA information can be obtained
at www.ICGtesting.com
Printed in the USA
LVHW022154271022
731749LV00002B/437